BIODYNAMICS OF OSTEOPATHY

Pediatrics One

Second Edition

James Jealous D.O.

For more information about Dr. Jealous please visit:
https://BiodynamicsOfOsteopathy.com

BIODYNAMICS OF OSTEOPATHY Pediatrics One

Hardback ISBN: 979-8-2955-3917-6

Second Edition 2025

James Jealous D.O. (1943–2021) practiced as an osteopathic physician, teacher and writer for many years. His life's work was to found and develop the specific methodology of Biodynamics of Osteopathy, following the lineage of Dr. A.T. Still and Dr. W.G. Sutherland.

This is one of a series of Biodynamics of Osteopathy books. They grew organically from sets of handouts written by Dr. Jealous and given to students during courses taught by him and his teachers. After many years he collected the handouts together and created individual course manuals, which he added to and rewrote many times. After several more years they evolved further into books.

TABLE OF CONTENTS

OSTEOPATHY IS SERVICE

We use our hands ...

To treat the Whole patient

To listen to the indwelling movements of Life

To treat all levels of illness

To assist in building the patient's functional reserve

To support homeostasis and trophicity by balancing the activity of the autonomic nervous system

To explore "laws not framed by human hands" (Dr. Still and Dr. Sutherland)

To cooperate and communicate with the Laws of Nature (Dr. Wales)

"To find the Health" (Dr. Still)

To get to the treatment plan

To get to the diagnosis

To help establish a point of Rest or Neutral around which the Whole can come to balance

To find Cause

We believe ...

We have an innate capacity to heal
The patient functions as a whole
The autonomic nervous system plays a major role in disease and healing
Structure and function are one form of activity
The Divine is indwelling
Life moves beyond death
There is a Constant Movement toward Normal
We are here to Serve Humanity

Normal is ...

"A sense of peace and harmony" (Dr. Sutherland)
Ease of motion, without tension
A capacity for Neutral
A sense of Wholeness to Life
The capacity for adaptation, change without compensation.

"Skill is proportionate to one's understanding of normal" (Dr. Still)

BIODYNAMICS ... WHERE DID IT COME FROM?

The name "Biodynamics" was chosen for a new curriculum in osteopathy because it was clear that many embryologists and Dr. Sutherland had much in common.

The story begins in 1966 with my first course in Sutherland's work. I was intrigued, but like any university-trained person, skeptical.

I graduated from Kirksville in 1970, after completing a fellowship in anatomy, did an internship, and went into rural practice as a GP. I made hospital rounds, delivered babies, made many house calls, and was on call most of the time. As an American D.O., I could prescribe drugs, but most of my care was osteopathically based. I used mostly functional technique, nutrition, and long conversations directed toward cause as the primary tools in practice.

Embracing skepticism, I set out to see if Magoun's book was accurate. Without reading the text, I listened to the cranium in search of Primary Respiration and involuntary tissue motions. Functional cranial work (indirect) was very helpful for my patients but I did not understand why it was so powerful. As a modest skeptic, I continued my research and was involved in mentoring students in my office constantly. Some of the students offered to help me with my proofs. We set out to dissect the dural system and get some good anatomy slides. The dissections challenged the three-sickle model. I began to research the growth and development of the dural system. In doing so I studied the 1978 Symposium on Development of the Basicranium from NIH. In these studies were descriptions of metabolic fields that behaved exactly like Sutherland's descriptions of fluid dynamics. I reread every word of Sutherland and began to read E. Blechschmidt's studies. After five years and piles of articles and books, I realized that Blechschmidt and Sutherland were discussing the same fluid. I then began to explore a premise that the embryological forces of growth and development are present throughout life as healing and sustaining metabolic processes. This premise is the foundation of Biodynamics.

When I applied the premise in treatments, the clinical results were much like what Sutherland said: "uncanny." My practice was overflowing with unexpected cures. Students pushed me for explanations and supported the project with dissections and study, often bringing articles that crescendoed our understanding.

Any understanding of anatomy as a metabolic movement changed my perception.

Is anatomy static or dynamic? How does the answer fit into a model of healing and repositioning? I reread Dr. Still's description of "what is anatomy" in *Philosophy of Osteopathy* (pages 16–19). There it was again, the same premise. In his case he saw it directly; I was climbing a steep hill toward his words with limited experience.

We continued to prove our premise in practice, that the embryological forces persisted throughout life. Younger physicians who worked with us gleaned the same remarkable results in their general practice.

Along the way some British osteopaths joined with us, and we formed a transatlantic study group that flourished with mutual respect and love. The friendship of fellow travelers, into an unknown uncharted sea, hastened the pace. The training began to take shape along with the realization that we could not condense 20 years of research and practice into 25 hours.

The courses began in 1990 as pieces, and formally in 1993. This is how the profession has grown ... mentors, students, professional friends and research that flow into practice. The proof is in the clinic; patients with all manner of disease are being seriously helped.

Embryologists are not feeling living systems; Sutherland was. There is, without a doubt, more about fluid dynamics to be learned from applied clinical osteopathy than from embryology. I say this not to create contrast, but to point out that our hands are listening to a system that creates living functions and sustains them. We are listening to nature at work.

We do not understand how, but we can learn to communicate and cooperate with metabolic expressions that become, with time, as familiar as any natural landscape. The indwelling therapeutic forces that Dr. Still knew well were coming alive.

As clinicians, our interest is in embryology in motion, its physiological wisdom.

THE MYSTERY OF FLUID DYNAMICS

Both Blechschmidt and Sutherland used their senses to observe fluid dynamics, Blechschmidt with a microscope, Sutherland with proprioception. Their outcomes were similar. If one compares their descriptions of fluid dynamics, one arrives at images that are exactly the same. Both describe fluid compression activities, expansion activities, opposing physiological motion activities, et cetera. Sutherland studied the fluid when it was still, in dynamic pauses, and when it was at work reorganizing lesion dysfunction. Sutherland saw that fluid could lesion, inhibiting osseous motion. This insight has far-reaching implications.

The problem of the nature of the "fluid" has been a dilemma for years. There are many reductionistic theories that have failed. The fluid is not water-like. It is protoplasmic in nature and therefore has a "livingness" that has a decision-making capacity. Both Blechschmidt and Sutherland observed this.

Protoplasm is the first moldable substance that can hold an image. Protoplasm becomes ectoderm, mesoderm, and endoderm. That sounds simple, except all the layers can become any of the other layers. The fact that the program is not set in stone, and has the capacity for transmutation, fits Sutherland's observations about fluid dynamics. He also saw that at Neutral all the fluid would interchange, resulting in powerful anti-inflammatory and transmutative phenomena. We have diverse bodily fluids arising from one fluid (protoplasm). The fact that protoplasm and its offspring can transmute raises more questions about the brain behind it all, because the CNS is not developed when this occurs.

Embryology points to an extra-genetic cause. Finding cause is an osteopathic principle. Cause is a mystery, a mystery of wholeness.

Wholeness is a living reality that creates the parts which are only an expression of the whole, nothing less. Parts are not the cause we are pointing at in osteopathy.

Fluid is not a fluid in the usual sense of the word; it is a symbol of fluency. Why the word "biodynamics"?

In all contexts this word points to a Mystery. Life dynamic. All of life as a "Whole Life." Blechschmidt was able to prove that there were extra-genetic forces at work in the unfolding of embryonic life as a wholeness. This means something beyond today's science.

Osteopathy as envisioned by Still recognized something he called Life. Again, a wholeness, not the sum of the parts. The action of wholeness is a Mystery. No one can capture it with instruments.

Blechschmidt states that something from outside the embryo influences its growth—a biodynamic principle. Still and Sutherland both sensed this principle. Sutherland actually asked his wife to paint a picture of a *House Under the Sea,* transparent to the motion of Primary Respiration. This was his summation of years of research. An outside force passing through us and creating and sustaining Life and our little life as we know it.

This Tide in the sea around and through us was called Primary Respiration. It was our most immediate environment. It influences all indwelling, healing, and sustaining forces.

"Biodynamic" equals a mystery, beyond "laws framed by human hands."

The similarities between Blechschmidt, Still, Sutherland, and their followers is something we can respect. They were all men of integrity and service. Sutherland began as a skeptic, which is healthy. We are all skeptics in a way, and that is how we learn to accept the Mystery.

Blechschmidt writes in *The Beginnings of Human Life* that "the Mystery is known only to the embryo" ...

This phrase touched me in a place that moves my whole quest for healing.

The innocent know the Mystery. The embryo, a pure and innocent whole, became an archetype for what Still called "the

Health," this sense of something perfect in oneself, veiled in secrecy, open only to neutrality and innocence. This set my heart on fire in a way I cannot explain ... nor can I explain the Mystery ... the Mystery has a sensation, a presence in every patient. From there comes a fire that sustains and heals.

A potency that transmutes exactly as Sutherland reported.

Biodynamics has grown by word of mouth. It has grown because it works in clinical practice. It has grown because we teach, knowing that what we know will change. Change is the hallmark of life; it is what we see under our hands. It is what we all hope for.

"Osteopathy is only in its infancy, it is a great unknown sea, just discovered, and as yet we are only acquainted with its shoretide."

(Philosophy of Osteopathy, preface, A. T. Still)

THE PHYSIOLOGICAL BASIS OF A BIODYNAMIC APPROACH IN THE CARE OF CHILDREN

Osteopathic thinking is the foundation of the approach.

Osteopathy is service; that is to say, there is no personal goal in the exchange with the patient.

In the 1978 Symposium on Development of the Basicranium, as well as the writings of Dr. Blechschmidt and Dr. Gasser, there are descriptions of metabolic fields that are exactly the same as Dr. Sutherland's descriptions of the fluid dynamics.

One can easily and comfortably conclude that the formative forces and intelligence that cause growth and development are present throughout life.

Is there any anatomy as we understand it? No?

Reread pages 16 to 19 in *Philosophy of Osteopathy*. What explains what one feels, that seems like anatomy?

One of Sutherland's most dramatic statements is "The fluid can lesion."

When fluid fields lesion from any cause, be it chemical, physiological, or physical, the metabolic dynamics "lock up," and one feels a form that is static, tense, rigid, congested, compressed, and isolated. The metabolic fields can have a huge range of motion, from ice-like to vapor. The nature of all metabolic tone comes from protoplasm, which has the range of being as described above.

The fluid behaves as a singularity, as one drop, as a wholeness that is indivisible whether lesioned or free. This reality is hard for us because we are focused on the parts, not the wholeness of the metabolic fields and life itself. Children live in this world, and any problem a child might have is in the interchanging with all the fluids of the body, not just one.

What causes healing, and what organizes growth and repair? It is not the brain!

What is the cause of the mechanism ... Where is the intelligence that organizes all this?

It is everywhere. The mind behind all of life is a mystery, but it is also concretely evident when we are silent and aware of this wholeness.

In a simple manner, we call the mind incarnate "the Health." The whole of the mind we call the "Beloved Mystery of Divine Love."

Children live in this mystery, and when approached through these principles they respond with familiarity.

When asked about cause, Dr. Blechschmidt said ...

"It is a mystery known only to the embryo. Think about this as you treat. Embryo ... health ... knowing ... Let the embryo speak with you."

PEDIATRICS ONE, THE HISTORY OF THE PEDIATRIC COURSES

The Convergence of the Teachings of A. T. Still, W. G. Sutherland, and Erich Blechschmidt. A Biodynamic Approach to Osteopathic Thinking and Treatment.

Dr. Still experienced osteopathy as the movement of life. Life itself could be partially experienced as mind (Divine), matter, and motion.

The mind of creation breathes through substance and creates motion. Motion is the essence of normal ... of health.

Chapter one, in the first edition of Magoun's *Osteopathy in the Cranial Field,* sums up Dr. Still's conclusions:

"Motion must be guided and directed by a supreme being down to the individual cell or there would be chaos and death." Dr. Still understood the cerebral spinal fluid as the highest known element in the human body. He envisioned this fluid as an intermediary in the movement of the divine intelligence ... a channeling of creation into embryological segments and irrigating them with life ... Giving form and function, order and intelligence to our existence. Without this there would be only decay and chaos.

In other words, motion created by a divine mystery unfolds itself in every form and function. The timing and orderliness of creation bear witness to this truth. In our work we can feel this motion as something passing through and suffusing everything with integrity and power, in a precisely detailed manner. Loss of the movement creates illness and, ultimately, death. The work of an osteopath is to support the continuum of this motion, which, when free, is self-organizing.

Dr. Sutherland reports his direct observation of the cerebral spinal fluid receiving the "Breath of Life." Dr. Sutherland felt a mysterious spark of unerring potency that was intelligent and in command, superseding all other function. This spark ignites wholeness.

Therefore he called it "Primary Respiration" because it was transcendent, quintessential, and "from the Fire."

Sutherland also observed that this motion of primary respiration organizes matter and orderly metabolic processes, while repairing dysfunction.

He sees the process as transmutation, not transformation.

He also noticed that this intelligence has diagnostic intention and priorities, and treats in a manner that is unerring in its skill.

He saw this potency as "working in a dynamic interchange with its own creation as one fluid."

To paraphrase: Sutherland sees the pattern of mind, matter, and motion collected, in the same manner as Still, and adds some language that brings into view more of the "feeling of fluid" that one gets during treatment; fluid moving through the fluid (the potency), something coming into the patient creating a change, great precision unfolding from a higher Mind; a great hidden mystery at work right down to every cell. Wholeness ... Self-correcting forces at work, and the indwelling capacity to heal. Form and function existing as a single form of being, embraced by creation and healing, as a mystery, all unfolding from eternity.

All of the foundational principles of osteopathy are laid out before us by both physicians. Their words reflect years of empirical science, years of watching and observing others. What made them famous was not their theories but the clinical results they gleaned. These are not ideas; rather, they are masterpieces of science, based upon and emerging from the art of practice. Patients came to them as physicians who treat all diseases, not just as neuromusculoskeletal medicine specialists! Read their case reports and you will see something remarkable. Understanding the principles that frame their work requires much time and effort.

The remarkable embryologist E. Blechschmidt brought to light truths that so parallel Sutherland that the coincidence itself is uncanny.

The root of osteopathy lies in embryological segmentation. These early localizations of function provide us with the schematic at the foundation of our interface with the autonomic and central nervous systems. Much has been written on this, and it is essential to our work.

The teaching on "the withering field" is based on this. Blechschmidt unveils a profound new view of metabolic fields that are the effects of a mysterious force, which synchronizes the process of growth and development as a whole. Order and precision so exact that he reports never seeing the indwelling intelligence miss the perfect geometric intersect.

He describes wholeness synchronizing segmentation. He also describes, with different words, the same fluid motions that Sutherland clarifies in his commentaries on fluid and "the fluid in the fluid."

Together, these works open our understanding to an ongoing drama, which validates much of what we feel during treatment.

It is not so much the milestones or sequences of growth that interest us, but the interplay of a mysterious intelligence, the fluid effects, and the synchronization of the parts in wholeness unfolding. Blechschmidt used the word "biodynamic" because of an interface between a supernatural outside force and the internal process. He leaves the Mystery as a secret known only to the embryo itself, as did Sutherland and Still. He sees this as a transcendent reality. But he also, like Sutherland, sees an internal process guided by the "biodynamic influence" as an automatic, precise, biokinetic activity; Sutherland, in viewing the same, called it "automatic shifting" (see 1953 *OCA Journal* article "Automatic Shifting").

In 1981 we began to ask the question ... Are the forces of growth and development the same forces present in primary respiration? Does this work in practice? After 10 more years of considerations on this, Biodynamics of Osteopathy was formally established as a postgraduate teaching program, put together by me with support from many wonderful friends. And to those who rejected our efforts, thank you for pushing us even harder in our attempt to be clear and precise in formulating this program.

Every effort has been made to use osteopathic language as Still and Sutherland used it because they are still teaching us. Sometimes the words do not work very well, but that is the legacy we carry...

We are grateful for the opportunity to share and learn more as we all unfold together.

In the 1949 *OCA Journal*, Dr. Sutherland wrote:

"I deem it my duty to caution in the usage of any application of direct action technique to the Basi-Sphenoid or Petrous Portion Apex.

"This type of technique directly affects (creates) a severe strain to the Junction of the Great Cerebral Vein with the Straight Sinus.

"Please consider this as a constructive criticism by one who has considerably more experience than most.....enough said I hope."

DIRECT AND INDIRECT ACTION IN THE OSTEOPATHIC TREATMENT OF CHILDREN

Most pediatrics courses teach direct action techniques ... that is, lesions are taken into the barrier in an attempt to engage therapeutics and reposition the bone in its proper anatomical position. Going to barrier does not allow the corrective forces of Primary Respiration or Thoracic Respiration to work unless at some point the barrier is consciously or unconsciously dismissed.

Direct action techniques tend to follow a line of thinking that is orthopedic; that is, that the displaced bone is entrapping a nerve and causing symptoms. This kind of reductionistic thinking engages the inertial barrier in the lesion, and not the Direction of Ease in the lesion. Indirect action techniques are the opposite. These principles exaggerate the permitted motion in the lesion (Direction of Ease), from which the name is derived. Still used both principles.

Direct action was promoted by Dr. Magoun and the American Sutherland Cranial Teaching Foundation (SCTF), because he felt that indirect technique was too hard for beginners; his reasoning, as reflected in his writings, is very biased toward direct action. However, indirect action is easier for most students because there is no force in the methodology. That relieves any fear of hurting the child. I believe there is wisdom in that.

Sutherland himself, when asked about direct and indirect action, preferred indirect (Lippincott, *A Manual of Cranial Technique*, page 1). The members of Sutherland's study group (circa 1939) were more fluid and indirect than Magoun, as is witnessed by reading the 1953 *OCA Journal.*

Why is this important?

First, you have a choice to make when you treat children ... and when you think about how they heal.

Second, there is a functional model that uses indirect, and a biomechanical model that uses direct. The end points are very different. The biomechanical end point is a local release, while the functional end point of a treatment is systemically cultivated.

Third, there is another method that we call biodynamic that does not use motion testing, but rather pursues the whole patient first, then the local motion present in the lesion field, then Neutral in the Whole and transmutation of tissue tension into a fluid field systemically. This method requires one to think independently of what one knows as a frame of reference, which is exciting.

Fourth, "think osteopathy" ... The whole, at a point of ease ... What is the easiest and quickest way to the desired end? What integrates your work once the treatment is in progress ... how can you prove it?

Children grow as a whole. Not in parts as we believe. Children live in the Direction of Ease of motion present in their fluid metabolic fields. Otherwise, they get uncomfortable and require assistance.

The only barrier they engage with is adult reductionism and tempo.

Growth is about being on time and at the right place. This process cannot happen without the wholeness expressing what we see as parts ... Wholeness is the essence of wellness, and in children this needs our thinking.

How does a normal child heal, or grow naturally?

Does your treatment directly support the whole, or does it assume to support the whole?

Reread *Philosophy of Osteopathy.* What was Still saying about anatomy, fluid exchange, wholeness, and the ease of fluid dynamics?

The following practical will involve direct, indirect, and

biodynamic methods, just so we can review the language of our profession and refresh our understanding of principles. How does one begin? What and when does the therapeutic force enter? What happens as a result of the therapeutic force, locally, systemically, and to you?

INDIRECT ACTION ON THE PELVIS

Practical

This is the first thing that Ruby Day, D.O., taught me. It comes from Dr. Sutherland.

With the patient sitting ... knees one inch free of the table to allow for automatic shifting ... place your hands under the pelvis so that the ischia are medial to your longest fingers.

Observe the pelvic bowl and pelvic floor.

The pelvic floor can be seen as the face of a clock ...

To find indirect method we motion test, clockwise and counterclockwise ... Which direction is easier? That is the Direction of Ease, or the indirect pathway to healing.

Move slowly into the Direction of Ease ... do not go too fast or you will hit resistance (i.e., barrier) ... the ease will come to a balance point where there is a sense of stillness and quiet ... This is called a Neutral ... the point where the therapeutic forces of thoracic and primary respiration can enter the lesion field and transmute the lesion. Just wait and a treatment will begin.

Your end point is when the pelvic bowl tissue responds to the breathing of Thoracic Respiration. There is an option for Primary Respiration's effect on the fluid field to be the end point.

TREATING THE PELVIS WITH BALANCED FLUID TENSION

We are focusing on the perinatal pelvis. This concerns the well-being of both the child and the mother.

The fluid we are concerned with is protoplasm. It is the basis of life. It is the vehicle from which all form and function emerge as a whole, on time and in the right place.

It can express a therapeutic event if Neutral is present, otherwise it may not perform accurately. The pelvic bowl is the same as the cranial bowl. It behaves in a similar fashion.

Compare the indirect and fluid approaches.

Listen to the fluid motion present.

Synchronize during the inhalation period.

Treatment.

End point.

•••

Recognition of the embryonic world.

THE CLINICAL HIGHLIGHTS OF TREATING THE PELVIS DURING PREGNANCY

The Prenatal Period

Please remember, we are not visualizing gross or segmental anatomy. Any mindset that goes after the lesion directly to release the somatic tension will fail to engage the power of the Dynamic Stillness, i.e., Primary Respiration.

Clinical results are proportionate to the application of principles that do not override the Tide and its wisdom. This demands discipline on your part; we must not apply biomechanical principles when using higher laws of healing. This is a hard thing for all of us to trust, but it will be worth the strife.

What you may see, without visualizing, are seams. These are the pre-segmental spatial dynamics of the protoplasmic matrix folding as a whole. During treatment, we often see an oval seam between the visceral and somatic components of the abdomen and pelvis as a single space.

Treatment from the pelvis changes the dynamics of the viscera (uterus, pelvic floor, prostate, bladder, gut, thoracic abdominal seam, etc.). During pregnancy, when the patients have adaptive symptoms such as urinary frequency, pyrosis, pelvic floor pain, and other functional problems, this approach really works ... easily.

The treatment feels like a warm gel molding; it ends in a Neutral. Be careful not to over-treat. If you do, you will get tired. The treatment takes place around the edges of the visceral sac and inside the somatic wall. Other types of activity are also possible. If you work this way prenatally, you will prevent fetal malposition.

Even if you do not deliver babies, you will still find that many people seek out treatment during pregnancy. As you treat some, more will come, because the treatments work.

If the patient does not come until the last weeks of pregnancy, you may think about using the "turning the baby" technique as well as the pelvic bowl approach, during the same visit.

If you read Dr. Still's comments on obstetrics, you will find enough osteopathic thinking to cure any orthopedic attitudes you might have picked up in your studies. Most health care professionals do not think osteopathically. We must claim our profession by living it. One of Still's strong suits is his awareness of the Whole as a reality.

In Dr. Still's description of balancing the pelvic floor (*Philosophy of Osteopathy*, section on obstetrics), he engages the "soft parts" above the pubes and the pelvic floor ... He says little ... If this plan is followed during the last trimester, you will feel the tissue become a gel. When we follow the "soft parts" as he suggests, the whole perineum is easily molded toward a new form (and no anatomy is felt). At the end point, the pelvis homogenizes ... then the movement of Thoracic Respiration empties itself through the pelvic floor. Something beautiful occurs, as a simple, deep Neutral emerges. This helps the bladder adapt and the cervix flatten, soften, and open.

Near the seventh month, another phenomenon occurs demonstrating the principle that "space opens in the Dynamic Stillness of the protoplasm and function moves in creating form." This is a fact of great importance. It is why we do not recommend trying to make the pelvis symmetrical by manipulating it.

During the middle of the third trimester, as you hold the pelvic bowl, you will feel a space inscribed in the fluid field that marks the space that is opening, as a passageway, into which the child can easily find a doorway through the pelvic floor ... As the child goes left or right it spirals around the midline, and when the head arrives in this world it is perfectly centered on the midline (sagittal suture centers on pubes). This is quite remarkable to witness--especially if you think birth is a mechanical interface between tissue forces, and that no preparation or transmutation is anticipated by Mother Nature and her friends.

Before labor, the head engages in a position that reflects the passage of the child in the Direction of Ease. As the child snuggles into position, the pelvic bones translate, and transmute, to meet the coming changes. They are not forced into a new "place"; rather, they synchronize with a known pathway and conform. The bones are breathing and molding along with the Tide, as is the child.

All these principles are quite beautiful. They are not created by science, but by nature. The Tide has healed our minds and senses to unveil something precious to us, and through that witness has come a tradition. The science of osteopathy.

During Labor

The movement of labor receives support and wisdom from many sources. The Long-Tide plays a role in setting the wholeness of the event in motion. It comes from the "sea around us," and in some mysterious way, catalyzes the ripening and transport of mother, child, and father into a new world. About a week before labor, the Long-Tide comes into the womb from the horizon and creates ignition. This fires labor.

If the parents are aware of these things, then it becomes spiritually fulfilling.

Newborns in the birth canal are able to "speak" with the mother; this guidance is necessary to appreciate the timing of events.

The movement in health care today is to think of pregnancy as something to get through, and then life, instead of becoming more, is forced to return to its prior pattern. The outcome is that the old pattern organizes a new form around the old fulcrum, and the immune system weakens. This requires us to educate the patient.

Labor should be supported by someone with insight and the time to commit to the event. Dr. Still believed that the osteopath should stay with the patient from the onset of labor to the end.

The treatment during labor is to have the patient sit, as in the practical. This position supports fetal momentum, and the mother can rest her arms on one of your shoulders. The treatment will be obvious as the forces of the Tide are extremely potent and focused.

The treatment is not routine. It is only necessary if some form of inertia enters the process. The mother will often find the position restful, and between contractions may rest on the Tide (looks like sleep).

Postnatal Treatment

The journey completes itself.

Now the forces that created the growth and change in the mother and child continue to work toward Wholeness. The child enters a new circle. We will discuss this elsewhere.

The mother has a large number of segmental, hormonal, mental, and visceral changes. The uterus, for example, must change size. It grew all the way up to the diaphragm (ovaries too). Now it returns to the pelvis. The peritoneal sac moved along with it. The Fluid Body opened all these changes before tissue transmuted. The shape of the head changed, the upper and lower leaves of the tentorium cerebelli moved dramatically, the pelvic floor turned gel-like, the breasts changed shape and content; the body fat content shifts, all the hormones move kaleidoscopically, the sense of self shifts, faith increases or decreases, the gut and bladder move around, the liver is busy, the placenta is gone, the immune system readjusts, the heart opens, then Zone B becomes communal ... all of the changes must find a single fulcrum as the mother moves into a new body and soul relationship ... treatment is helpful.

There are several highlights that I would like to note as places that need evaluation during the immediate postpartum period.

As was noted above, the tents change during pregnancy. If they do not unfold after delivery, the patient can have thyroid dysfunction, headaches, mild hypertension, etc. The principle is treatment of the Whole, but if that is not forthcoming easily then one can go to the seam between tents and find the Long-Tide, as we did in Phase Three. The treatment is simple, so do not hang out too long trying to fix tissue or you will miss the fruit. Once the treatment starts, there is no anatomy, unless one is not allowing the Tide to center them.

The results are immediate (48 hours or less). Remember that the core of the hormonal system is at the fulcrum of the tents' origin, and they develop as one movement. As the Long-Tide works, it moves everything. That is why, once the treatment starts, no anatomy is visible.

The next place to evaluate, if the Whole will not respond, is the thoracic–abdominal seam. This seam is the point of interface between the thorax and the abdominal cavities. Work here rebalances the functional synchronicity between the peritoneal sac, the diaphragm, the esophagus, etc.

The symptoms that arise if this area needs to be addressed could be constipation, referred shoulder and neck pain (common), postpartum uterine bleeding (mild, persistent), nausea, pyrosis, and dysmenorrhea.

If this is not addressed, many years later the patient will become short-waisted and even develop mild hypertension or idiopathic edema of the lower limbs due to pressure on the adrenal–renal area and lymphatics. Looking at this seam can be helpful for the whole visceral tree. The treatment follows the same principles as those described for the tents. However, by now you realize that the Tide will move from one level of treatment to another. If we begin in a seam with the presence of the Long-Tide, then we may end up in deeper water.

Rebalancing after each treatment is advisable.

The treatment of the mother/child/father as one is covered

elsewhere. Treatment of children is a separate course because the principles are unique.

THE PRENATAL PELVIS

Osteopathy can prevent many hardships for children as they enter this world.

The first line of prevention is the state of the maternal pelvis and its capacity for change. The bones, ligaments, and muscles need to transmute from muscle tissue to a gel-like state. This should be recognizable the last month and progress thereafter.

Treatment during pregnancy using biodynamic principles supports the metabolic changes that allow the muscles to soften into a gel. It is quite remarkable. This is easily felt during treatment of the perineum in the last month of pregnancy. The evaluation for these changes is done as Still advises in *Philosophy of Osteopathy.* One hand is placed above the pubes on the soft parts, and one below on the soft parts of the perineum. What one feels is a gel ... not soft muscles ... this gel-like state of the muscles means that the pelvis is preparing for birthing. The gel-like state almost obliterates fascial planes, evident in a nonpregnant pelvis. The treatment is therefore not BMT, but BFT, balanced fluid tension.

Seeing these changes should remove some of the illusions that labor is a "mechanical war" between the uterus, the child, and the pelvis. Mother Nature knows what's coming and prepares a Direction of Ease. We need to make sure that the patient is able to express these changes of the tissues becoming fluid. If this is not occurring then we must treat the whole Fluid Body that mediates these changes.

THE PASSAGEWAY

One expression that sums up the process of birthing is this: Space opens in the fluid, and function moves into the space that opens. By the eighth month, if one senses the fluid field of the pelvis, there will be an opening, a space shaped like a spiraling tube. It will be either left or right of center. It is the passageway prepared for the child to move along as labor begins. The child's physical position should match this space. This shape is the real birth canal, so to speak. Knowing what is happening allows one to predict the movement of the child as ROA, LOA, etc.

Again we see Mother Nature being fully prepared to create an amazing process.

This passageway is a space in the fluid, not a musculoskeletal positional shift. It has the shape of a tunnel from the pelvic rim to the pelvic floor. The pelvic tissues will shift afterwards to follow the space and its shape in exactly the same manner in which embryonic growth and development proceed. In other words, space opens, and function moves in.

Do not try to symmetrize the pregnant pelvis or you will inhibit this process, which is asymmetrical.

FETAL MALPOSITION, TURNING BABIES

If the pelvis is treated during pregnancy, fetal malposition is preventable. We will discuss this.

Fetal malposition is treatable without any direct action techniques, either manual or with straps. This sounds crazy. In 1982 when I began teaching how to turn babies, there were many raised eyebrows. Since then thousands of babies have been successfully turned using a simple principle of treatment. The treatment is safe, easy to accomplish, and follows the principles of osteopathy completely. All of the babies that I am aware of from multiple sources were turned in the last few weeks before labor. All types of fetal malposition, from transverse lies to breech, have responded to treatment.

Three percent of the cases fail to reposition. We have followed the delivery histories on some of the "failures." In most cases the cord was around the neck in such a manner that turning may have been traumatic for the child.

Because no force is applied, the safety of this procedure is wonderful.

Why the baby turns is a Mystery of Nature. We have learned a lot in 25 years. But the principle has not changed since its beginning in 1982. The truth of an indwelling movement toward normal is validated over and over again ... this capacity to reposition around a midline is a natural occurrence in the realms of Primary Respiration. There is plenty of science that points to repositioning as a possibility. However, our mechanistic formats resist these truths, even when stated by experts in both embryology and osteopathy ... All I can say is, try the principles and see for yourself.

A Story

In 1979 a patient came to see me. She was a pediatric nurse who had been a patient before, as had some of her family members. She was at eight and a half months with her second child. The baby was in a transverse lie ... her first child was also transverse and had to be forcibly turned.

She was distraught at the idea of another forceful procedure. "Dr. Jealous, I want you to turn my baby," she said. I was shocked at her request. "I do not know how," I said. "Yes, you do," she said. "I have seen you do many unexpected things for your patients."

I resisted her commentary, and she persisted ... after several go-rounds with her I decided to center the uterus around its original midline and wait. I did nothing to the child.

I laid her on her side facing me ... the fundus of the uterus was lying on the table and the cervical os was higher up ... so that the uterus and the passenger were downhill from the pelvis.

I knew the uterus had a midline, so I lifted the fundus until the uterus and passenger were level (as with a carpenter's level). As the pregnant uterus "leveled," the patient involuntarily rolled a little toward me. I let her come, and as she did I followed the Direction of Ease with her. The uterus wanted to go toward the spine ... so we went, without any barrier ... there came a sense of centering. I waited (out of ignorance) ... she then sat up! I was certain I had done nothing ... at no time did I feel the uterus or passenger move ... it was quiet, if anything.

She called the next day and the baby had turned during the night ... she was sure that the cause was osteopathy! I was rethinking the whole event ... just in case there was a principle at work that I needed to recognize ... I tried turning another child, and it worked ... then others tried it. The results are wonderful.

Since then, children worldwide have been turned using this technique of centering the uterus on its midline ... it is hard to believe it until you do it ... the science of osteopathy comes out of the art of osteopathy. I became more aware of the magnitude of what we do not know, and how we must always "think osteopathy" and give it a chance to show itself to us, as it did to Dr. Still.

Homework

Study the embryological development of the uterus ... just look at the pictures and see the two primordia meet ... they journey, as the Whole, toward a destination that already exists, in an invisible matrix of perfect geometry that was laid down at conception ... the two halves of the uterus come together around a midline (not shown in embryology texts) and center themselves upon it ... The two become one. The cervical os is on the midline, as is the apex of the fundus ... It all seems obvious to me ... if it seems questionable to you, we can review some facts from embryologists, who see this precision as perfectly as did Sutherland.

The pregnant uterus has a midline, and the child obviously spirals around it as it births.

My sense of fetal malposition is that it is caused by a loss of midline orientation, either by the uterus (mother), the child, or both as a singularity. I sense that the mother and child share the same midline in totality ... This central midline is not in the books.

It is an understanding developed from working with elders and my own experience using Fluid Body dynamics as a primary approach. All of it is based on Sutherland's sense of direction. It is worth pondering!

A REPORT ON FETAL MALPOSITION

I have been following "C" during her pregnancy on a regular basis. Her physician diagnosed depression and wanted her to take antidepressants, but she refused and was coming for osteopathic treatment at a rate that she determined, which was quite often. In the previous months, I really saw her getting happier and happier. A few weeks ago, her physician observed that the baby was positioned transversely. She planned an external cephalic version at the hospital for last Friday (week 37 of pregnancy). C was unable to come for osteopathic treatment until Thursday, the day before the ECV. As I thought this was a very short time for the body to equilibrate itself, I suggested that C go see an acupuncturist, which she did three days before her osteopathic appointment.

On Thursday, as she entered the office, I observed that her belly had a diagonal shape, from the top right quadrant to the bottom left quadrant. C lay down on the table, but she really had a huge difficulty coming to any form of Neutral. Coming to Neutral was difficult throughout the pregnancy; imagine one day before this intervention. As I was trying to help her go to a Neutral, I remembered the lab we did in Pediatrics 2: synchronization of the Thoracic Respiration with the Primary Respiration. So I helped C visualize her respiration. She calmed down and was able to attain a great, profound third-level Neutral. I positioned myself with one hand on the uterus and one on the lumbar spine.

Soon I witnessed a beautiful light creating a oneness, a Whole, engulfing mother and child. For once they were able to meet in a faraway place … tuned in, together … C rested on the table for a while after. When she was ready, she shared with me her experience. She was deeply impressed by the great feeling of love that she felt. I think that she experienced this for the first time. We discussed that whatever the issue of the version the next day, with that kind of harmony things could only turn out to be the best for both mother and child. When she left my office, her uterus was centered with her body.

C left a message for me on the phone at the end of the day Friday. Here is what happened. She arrived at the hospital in the morning. Her physician did an echographic exam; the baby was still transverse, but his head was now on the top left side (more diagonal than transverse). She had to wait, under medical supervision, for the arrival of the obstetrician. After a while, she felt tremendous pain. She almost fainted and said everyone was scared. It passed. When the obstetrician arrived to do the manipulation on the baby ... he was already head down, feet up.

Amen.

A NORMAL CHILD

Children are a living dynamic, not a static structure.

Children are never the same for two days in a row ... any patient observer can see this ... they change ... this is true of the consciousness as well as the soma.

This ever-changing form is not the addition of substance to an anatomical infrastructure that expands ... rather, the changes occur as the old form dies, and the new form is printed in the Fluid Body, after which the tissues fall into a form created by the intelligence behind creation and unfoldment ... The change is metabolic, and the unfolding form is the Health ... Both are guided by a mysterious force we call Primary Respiration. The chemistry and histology move as one Wholeness.

Death powers growth ... The old is transmuted, and a new form unfolds from the blueprint of life, established at conception. This moving blueprint is the basis of pediatric milestones.

These processes go on throughout our lifetime; they do not end with the embryo or the maturation process.

This premise wed to Sutherland's work in embryology was the beginning of a biodynamic model in 1982.

"Children Are Little Balls of Silence"

Max Picard, The World of Silence

IMAGES OF THE HEALTH, FROM STILL AND SUTHERLAND

Children are transparent to the Health.

These words are paramount to the treatment of children, in the Biodynamic Method.

Certainly Dr. Still posed a very profound truth when he said, "Find the Health; anyone can find disease." ... What does this mean? ... What is it like to experience the Health in oneself and others? ... Has anyone described it?

Drs. Still and Sutherland both describe experiences of the Health.

At the age of eighty-six, Dr. Still said, "I love my patients, I see God in their faces and their form."

These words are not timid. Dr. Still was straightforward. He was not looking at lesions. How did he come to this "ability"?

I can report on how this has happened for thousands of osteopaths, and myself—practitioners who do see the Health, the Divine, and a movement of life in their patients.

My introduction was from Dr. Becker personally, and in his 1965 Sutherland Memorial Lecture about the Spiritual Fulcrum. He states, "The Deity centers us." This refers to the Divine centering us ... not we centering ourselves. This awareness is common in contemplative practices that appreciate our inner poverty; "it is by the grace of God that we can perceive the invisible work of the Spirit." There is a distinct awareness when this happens to us. We are transformed in seconds to being an effect of another deeply loving presence. Our effort must have ceased in order for us to see the moment of impregnation and a total change in being.

Still was clear that human intelligence has severe limits without the intercession of a higher mind.

To witness the Health in another person, one's senses must be transmuted by the Health touching one's being when one is Neutral. This was made clear to me by Rollin when he looked at me one day and said, "Do not begin your treatment until the will of the patient surrenders to the will of Primary Respiration!" He was very direct and concrete as he said this. I was shocked. *He had taken the end point of treatment as I understood it and made it the beginning.* After many years his guidance became clear and profound.

The treatment begins when there is a sustained Neutral in the Whole. Children have this most of the time. Even sick children are transparent to the Health. This transparency is a special kind of Neutral that is persistent in children in spite of their disease. *Children do not lose their capacity to love, even when they are critically ill.* Adults, as you know, change their moods with their sense of wellness. *You will find that even very ill children will center you.* They transmit the flow of the Divine.

When we are in a Neutral that is saturated with Third Level Stillness, we become receptive in a unique manner. We are Neutral, waiting serenely for the Tide to enter the moment and unveil the senses to the invisible world of the Health. This is the Deity centering us, creating a new level of awareness ... In working with children, because they are deeply suffused by the Divine and the incarnate Health, their mere presence is enough to "center" us and bring our senses to "seeing" the Health ... if ...

we are Neutral and at the "Meeting Place," that is, the Third Level of Stillness.

This requires a certain inner awareness of the many ways we can fool ourselves.

As we are, our senses operate from the self-centered mind of our self-image. What does this mean? The synapses in our brain develop around familial and cultural interchanges. As children and young adults, we have many projections placed on us. From these trillions of synapses, we form a synthetic center ... one we create from the world around us, not the one in us from the beginning of Life. Many of us are working to "find our Health and discover ourselves" as we were originally made. That is to say, "to see God's face and form in ourselves and others," as Dr. Still stated.

Our senses are attached to the ego, and so we see others as projections of our own classifications, not as transparent beings reflecting the Divine image of the Health. We are all doing this. This understanding helps us to understand Neutrality and to make a choice to allow Deity to center us ...

Children will do this for us ...

if we meet them at the Meeting Place.

The transparency of a child to the Health allows the Health to come out into the world, and those who are able will respond by being "centered by the child" ... then we are able to see the Health in others. This is the first principle of treatment in this course.

One sees the world as transparent and whole. The sense we have of a child is that they are "empty" and transparent to the movement of creation. We see a transcendent love entering through them, creating/healing the cellular unfoldment of the child.

This appreciation of a simple and clear awareness of creation is part of the legacy we receive from Drs. Still and Sutherland. Let's review their teachings.

Dr. Still refers to mind/motion/matter.

Dr. Still said that these laws are not "framed by human hands."

The mind he speaks of is the Supreme Intelligence of the Divine Mystery. This Mystery animates as the Breath of Life (i.e., motion) which incarnates as the material world (matter). Thus we have Spirit moving into creation and unfolding the blueprint of life. We can see this if we are "centered by the Tide." When centered, we can see mind, motion, and creation as a singularity in the movement of life as a Whole.

The sensation of eternity entering time is beauty.
Sutherland and others follow the lead of Still.

In the first edition of Magoun's *Osteopathy in the Cranial Field,* Sutherland reports both his and Still's view of the Health:

A transparent Wholeness without systems or parts.

Remember, this is not philosophy, but the report of direct perceptual activity.

"... Motion must be guided by a Supreme Being, down to the individual cell, otherwise there would be chaos and death." (A. T. Still)

Sutherland then quotes Still further:

"Dr. Still understood the Cerebral Spinal Fluid as the highest known element in the human body; he envisioned this fluid as an intermediary in the movement of Divine Intelligence ... A channeling of Creation into embryological segments and irrigating them with Life ... giving ... form and function, order and intelligence to our existence. All Life is manifest in his Motion" (see page 15, paragraphs 1 and 2) ... awaken to the Health and you will witness this.

In *Contributions of Thought,* Sutherland again addresses a simple picture of Wholeness (see April 12th, 1948):

Here Sutherland describes feeling the cerebral spinal fluid (CSF) and the Breath of Life, the movement of Supreme Intelligence ... feeling the spark of life that ignites the potency. An unerring, overshadowing, and superseding function that he called Primary Respiration.

He sees a dynamic interchange (Becker) between creation and the created…

These impressions came to Sutherland only after he stopped using force!

Later in life Dr. Sutherland asked his wife to paint a picture of Primary Respiration, as he experienced it. Again another image appears that mimics those we have just discussed: a house under the sea.

The painting was lost in political bickering, but the story has been told to me by three of my mentors: Ruby Day, Anne Wales, and John Harakal. Recently, I was told by a historian that the house in the painting was A. T. Still's cabin … That would suggest a very deep love and remembrance of his teacher.

The House Under the Sea is biodynamic, in the sense that this image is similar to Blechschmidt's insistence that we are formed from a mysterious force, coming through us from the "outside." The similarity with Still, Sutherland, and the foundation of osteopathy in embryology is what prompted me to choose the name The Biodynamics of Osteopathy. The commonality of images provoked by all these observant men is heartwarming to anyone who has felt these things and feels a little crazy when told there is only structure in osteopathic diagnosis and treatment.

The image of a house, transparent to the ocean of the Breath of Life, brings again the sensory experience of transparency, of "something" passing through us, unimpeded, that heals/creates as it passes, without diminishing itself. This Supreme Intelligence is the Master Mechanic, the Physician Within, The Health, The Higher Self, and the Divine Image in all of Life…

Children are the Archetype of Normality, Radiant with these Truths.

Our elders saw these truths ... we can approach their teaching only when we are Neutral and free to be centered by Deity ... This is why we call it "The Meeting Place." The 1949 lecture of Dr. Sutherland teaching "the Tide" clarifies this in another manner.

We will learn how to let the child communicate with us, and from this, see into the therapeutics that are so different from adults, and so beautiful.

"I am not ashamed to be a child in the mind of God" (A. T. Still).

What is a child?

What does it feel like to be a child in the mind of God?

Are children aware of the movement of their own creation/creator? What does a child see, hear, taste, and smell?

What touches them?

When they see adults, what do they see in them?

Dictionaries fail to truly define a child.

Psychology is still pondering as to whether their perception is illusion or reality.

Most mothers understand that children see with love, a transcendent love, an unconditional love.

Many see children as in need of adult dogmas and restraints in order to grow up. Few believe that growth and development is extra-genetic and self-manifesting.

However, the principles of osteopathy state that a great Mystery is unfolding in a child, and is well guided by creation.

This is our place of orientation in this teaching ... so let's begin!

COMMUNICATION WITH CHILDREN

As we begin the study of communication with children, we explore the idea that they will center us by their transparency to the Health. A radiance flows through them. They are not pretending to be anyone. They are innocent of their beauty. The radiant flow touches us, and our senses reconnect to the Health in us. We begin to see new landscapes.

The idea of being centered by an outside source is foreign to most people. The process of dependency upon a higher mind than one's own seems like a nice idea, but the reality is that we are trained to resist changes not governed or understood by our will/ego complex.

In order to be healed by the child, so that our senses are realigned with the Health and we consequently can diagnose and treat in a deeper manner, we must be still and neutral so that the therapeutic force can shift our state of being. Being internally quiet is not an act of suppression of the emotions and thoughts that come into our awareness ... It is a Neutrality ... a state that is not active or passive ... it is a place you can experience.

Let's do a meditation and see if we discern different levels of activity in ourselves: Imagine that inside you is a deep well. At the bottom is the perfect Health.

But ... the well appears to be dark, and so the depth is not predictable. Let us explore these depths using the question,

What is a child?

–The intellect, or rational mind, is at the top of the well ... superficially, what is a child, what do most people think a child is? Think about a definition.

Now drop down in the well a little.

–The acquired intuitive mind will feel the question differently. What is a child? ... Wait in the well at this level.

Now drop down in the well a little more.

–The instinctual mind is connected with Nature herself. Ask again at this deeper place, what is a child? Wait ... Go further down into the darkness ... if you wish ... take the question with you.

–When you come to an empty room with "no mind," you are at the Meeting Place.

–We will now repeat the exercise, with our hands on the patient. Just wait for the Health in the patient to change you, as you wait at the Meeting Place.

What Is a Child?

Think logically, rationally ... pause ... what does your mind answer? Now let the question drop down into the intuition or the heart ... does the answer take a different form?

Let's drop down inside ourselves a little further, into a quiet room; close the door and sit in the question, without words or feelings ... pause ... what kind of knowing comes ... how does it differ from the first and second answers? Do you recollect your childhood mind?

Where is it now ... silenced?

Is there a meeting place where you can sense this childlike mind in yourself? ...

Go back into that room that is deep inside and just wait ... what transpires ... this is the Meeting Place.

The first principle of treatment is to wait in this "meeting place" ... until your awareness is changed by something that happens to you, not something that you do or make happen. One waits ... nothing more ...

How is communication established with the Health and consciousness in a child?

If we wait at the Meeting Place, the child's presence will have an effect on our awareness. Your consciousness is remarkably elevated and transparent, and the kinds of things that W. G. Sutherland and A. T. Still have spoken about will enter your perception ... here you begin the challenge of not falling back into old forms of being.

Let the love suffuse your awareness ... hold onto the change in your heart and mind even if your mental wheels turn away ... this is the beginning of communication and seeing the movements of creation. We come to a meeting place, the child greets us, we change, and we now begin to take a small step into the world of a child.

Practical: Go to the meeting place, level three, what transpires?

Learn to know yourself and be merciful ...

Do not push away undesirables in yourself ...

Stay in the Direction of Ease in your awareness.

What happens?

"I love my fellow man. I see God in his face and in his form."

A. T. Still, age 86

THE PERCEPTUAL JOURNEY TO THE MEETING PLACE

–Habit sets us in a direction
–Abreaction (away from habit)
–New landscape appears

–Waiting

–Landscape reveals its dimensionality
–Detachment (this is a choice to move toward the perfect in all of us; the Health)
–Wait … empty … not passive!

–Neutrality

SOMETHING converts your consciousness.
Awareness of health, transparency, and peace

THE SCIENCE OF GROWTH AND THE FLUID BODY

Once we came to understand the Fluid Body and its perfect intelligence, we began to realize that children are not adults. This sounds absurd to say, but the approach that was and often still is accepted as the standard for osteopathic treatment of children is direct confrontation of a lesion barrier with force directed by the physician.

This is in direct contradiction to the work that Sutherland prescribed later in his career.

Putting that aside, one is still faced with the facts that the physiological basis of growth and development, as well as Sutherland's observations of the "Fluid," both clearly point us away from a biomechanical approach as a first choice for treatment.

Growth and development is an expression of a unified protoplasmic syncytium, which is governed by an unerring mysterious force. The wholeness of a child is the smallest division ... This fact is expressed by modern embryologists as well as Sutherland. Dr. Still points in this direction in the opening chapters of *Philosophy of Osteopathy*. This must be addressed and integrated as we explore the responsibility of helping children become more normal.

As the whole changes shape and chemistry, there is, of necessity, the "death of the old" and the "unfolding of the new." This is how growth occurs. The old dies and the new informs. We are not piling up layers like a tree. This metabolic process is guided by Primary Respiration. The blueprint of life is unfolded, a story that is indwelling from conception. It is accomplished by transmutation.

Unfolding depends upon timing and position ... both are expressed in protoplasm while the whole is moving around a fulcrum ... a point of power and spatial dynamics.

The idea of position as a static anatomical place is so erroneous that I wonder how we missed this point earlier. There is a form that is changing its position, volume, and chemistry as we sit and treat. It happens now, not later.

This biodynamic syncytium must express its power as a whole, otherwise there will be system failures ... failures that, left to wither, will lead to gross disease patterns and morbidity. This is mainstream science, and however neglected it is ... we are the only profession that has the skills to interface with this marvelous and mysterious beauty.

Our task is to test the principles that co-emerge from these sciences and see where that leads us in the treatment of children. We must learn to communicate and cooperate with the natural laws at work by letting them teach us. And as I said ... think osteopathy!

Personally, I began the process of probing the principles in 1978. I mention this because I did not trust the material Sutherland proposed. But I love osteopathy, and the little effort I made paid incredible dividends in the clinical outcomes of my rural general practice.

I was sure that the results I saw were not true even when they stared me in the face. How could someone heal if the motion in the patient was addressed instead of the lesion tensions? It is hard to accept what you will see and feel and demonstrate in healing. The science exists, but it's too beautiful to be true. It is easy to write it off or say that we need force in hard cases.

What I have learned from being a GP and walking the line between allopathic and osteopathic medicine is that how one thinks will determine the principles one uses in practice. An allopathic mind doing osteopathy is doomed to use direct mechanical pressure or add remedies ... but if one can think differently about one case a week, the outcomes will prove the principles of osteopathy to that person.

Be a scientist and test the principles we set forth here, and you will discover why we are a distinct profession.

Children are biologically moldable and plastic … They are not adults, and coming to understand who and what they are is our purpose in studying.

If you treat an adult as a child, you will find that the laws of healing never change with age.

"You cannot treat a child as an adult, but you can treat an adult as a child."

WHOLENESS

Wholeness is the smallest division of life. The parts are expressions of the whole. There is no migration in growth, only the whole changing as singular form.

The idea and perception of Wholeness is not new in osteopathy, but it is often taken as a philosophical truth, not as a biological fact. Whole is a fact, and both Still and Sutherland came to appreciate Wholeness. As we treat children and pregnant mothers this fact is paramount, not just an idea ...

Zone B is a name given to the Fluid Body ... as we shall see, it acts as one drop without any distance. When shock of any nature occurs, the Fluid Body "breaks and deforms," aligning itself with a false midline rather than the one in the blueprint of the Health ... in children, this lesioning of the Fluid Body causes many delays and deformities. Restoration of the Fluid Body repositions all functions to a more perfect midline. Pediatrics One will work with principles that restore Wholeness.

Axioms

Growth and development are expressions of Wholeness.

The movement of Wholeness is perfect, in both its outcome and its capacity to reorganize itself if impeded. This is the creative concern of life for itself. It moves every molecule in perfect timing, creating effects we call milestones ... the perfect intersect of being, form, and expression.

Being, form, and expression are one movement. If lesioned, Wholeness partitions itself into what we call tissue, fluid, and potency. Normally these partitions are not felt in a healthy child or adult.

The blueprint of the Health does not lesion ... only the Fluid Body that has been genetically modified from the blueprint can deform.

MAMMALIAN EMBRYOGENENSIS

Evidence that some events of mammalian embryogenesis can result from differential growth, making migration unnecessary

"As a principle of physics, all movements occur in relation to a reference point. This is especially important in an expanding mass, such as an embryo, since all structures not attached to the surface understandably move away from the surface as the mass expands. Under such conditions, the ideal reference point would be one in the center of the mass, i.e., a centroid. Even though no such consistently occurring point exists in developing embryos, any point that is more centrally located would move less in relation to surrounding structures and therefore would be more suitable. Such reference points were used in the present study and differ from the surface or near-surface reference points used in past experimental studies on migratory movements."

Raymond F. Gasser PhD

The full article can be found here: https://anatomypubs.onlinelibrary.wiley.com/doi/full/10.1002/ar.b.20092

ZONES AS A TEACHING TOOL

Zones are a teaching tool that we have developed for Biodynamics.

Zone A is the somatic tensions that cannot become Neutral (rest).

Zone B is the protoplasmic field that can lesion.

Zone C is the operator's awareness of Wholeness in any form.

Zone D is the ocean between us and the horizon ... the biodynamic cause of Zone B

A normal child has no zones ... they feel TRANSPARENT

QUOTES FROM SEVEN TO NINE YEAR OLD CHILDREN

In 1979, a dance teacher from New York, who summered in rural Maine, told me that during her treatments she could feel the warm fluid movements. This occurred on a regular basis after she had her first three treatments. She taught children to dance and express fluidity in motion. She said she wondered if children could naturally feel what we call Primary Respiration.

She set up an experiment. She asked the children to feel inside themselves and report. Nothing more was said to the children.

1. It felt like a sea of people that were fighting over me. (Joana, grade 3)

2. My imagination works with the whole body and looks like crawling on grass. (Jason, grade 4)

3. Mine looks like a brain, feels like a big circle in my head. (JoAnn, grade 2)

4. My imagination is like a blob. It changes shape, size, and color. If you could feel it, it would feel slippery and spongy. It scoops up ideas and squeezes them into one idea. It fixes it up so that it is as good as can be and sends it to my mind. My mind sends it to my hands, and I do it. (Alon, grade 4)

5. It felt like someone was in a boat. It felt like I was in a boat. (Daniel, grade 3)

6. My imagination changes by the minute. Now it's in my stomach. (Jacob, grade 2)

7. Opening and closing. (Ryan, grade 2)

8. My mind has many thoughts. Today her thought is a bird. Not just any bird though! (Erin, grade 4)

9. Blue fire, fierce fire. (Daniel, grade 4)

10. I can't go inside my mind without going side to side. It's so windy. I find out that the wind is wavy, and it has special vitamins to pick up things. (Renee, grade 3)

11. If it is trapped, it feels like it is going to die. (Amy, grade 4)

12. Wee-hee-hee-hee-hee-hee. (Keith, grade 4)

13. It wants to be free. It doesn't want to be in an enclosed area. It likes to just be a nice summer breeze. (Jennifer, grade 4)

14. Freedom! (Nicholas, grade 4)

15. Very, very, wavy. (Angela, grade 4)

16. It feels like there is a bunch of water in my head spinning around. It feels like firemen are praying water in my head. (JB, age 7)

If children can feel the "Fluid Body" and observe it, then we must be careful to realize and honor their sensibilities and natural gifts. Children are invaded by many good intentions… Therefore, education of ourselves and parents is important.

MEETING WITH CHILDREN, BEING CENTERED BY THE CHILD

The goal of an osteopathic treatment is to find the Health in the patient, in such a manner as to let them choose to be reconnected with their Wholeness and the consequent somatic sensation of Eternity and Love.

With adult patients, we follow the leadership of Primary Respiration through landscapes that become familiar to us over a period of time. We have, to a greater or lesser degree, become familiar enough to cooperate and communicate with the laws that organize these landscapes. We can take some leadership in giving advice, should we be asked.

Children are not adults ... at all.

Our research with children and how to meet them has increased the success of clinical outcomes by such a great degree that comparison with our "older style of treatment" is of no benefit at all.

How do we enter the landscapes that children live in? What therapeutic format does Primary Respiration utilize, if we cannot inhibit the process? To answer the question directly, you can watch children play, fall down, and self-treat by stopping and being still, as a potent and soft substance fills them and leaves in several seconds. Or you can watch a mother hold an injured child and pray silently, expecting the grace of God to intervene and heal ... which it does.

Unfortunately, few people in modern society sense either event.

As osteopaths we may be able to follow the above activities, but only if our senses have been reconnected to a neutral mind ... Being active with the senses blinds us to these things, as does being passive or afferent. Neutral senses are connected to the Health. This is not an act of "will" but rather the outcome of being centered by a higher Mind, as Still and his followers have stated.

Children are with their Health in a manner that shames any adult who has noticed that even the most seriously ill kids can love beyond anything adults in general transmit. Adults, as you know, are not transmitting love in an unimpeded flow ... as a matter of fact, most adults are hostile to their illness and rarely feel this love, which is so familiar to children that they do not identify with it as "other."

Meeting children in a childlike manner is a good doorway to social contact. But that is not what is needed to understand the landscapes of the healing forces in a child, when the treatment begins and ends, and its style of potency and fire.

Can we become a child? Not in the sense we hope for. Treatments usually transcend our adult humanity and spiritual maturity ... so we will often be left behind in a place that we feel is paradise as the child moves ahead, behind another veil.

The Meeting Place is the place where we can begin to enter the lower edges of a child's world. A place they will recognize as shelter and safety. A place their parents occasionally visit with them, but perhaps not with intention or much frequency. Their response will prove what we say here, and will, I presume, impress you in many ways.

The Meeting Place occurs at the circumference of the Dynamic or Third Level Stillness.

THE DYNAMIC STILLNESS

The language used here is to highlight specific qualities of this unique Stillness. The multiple names are used in different areas of the teaching of Biodynamics of Osteopathy, where the emphasis shifts to detailed study of specific clinical circumstances.

The names for this Stillness are Third Level Stillness, Natural Stillness, Meeting Place, and Dynamic Stillness.

In our work we meet many kinds of stillness and stillpoints, with varying degrees of depth and power (potency). Each name refers to a particular kind of potency.

Third Level Stillness is intrinsic to undisturbed natural environments.

In the wilderness there are no roads. There are no psychic influences from the frenzy of civilized activities. The natural world is minimally changed by civilization in a wilderness area.

This Third Level Stillness is so strong that it overshadows all sounds; even the movements of animals and weather do not drown it out. It rules the sensory world.

It echoes immortality and frees the heart from any concern of death being a black hole. It is a food and a tonic that strengthens all the atrophy. It hardens the bones.

If one is thrown into a landscape with Third Level Stillness, its power can seem overwhelming. It frightens many early visitors. Once we are used to its presence, it is strong, stable, and supportive. It centers us. It holds us on its center. There is no work to do, other than respond to the movements of life. If one adores this place, then other qualities become known. It is not a place for persons who are not interested in spiritual death and the Health.

As we go along paved roads, there are some "out-of-the-way places" where this Third Level Stillness can be found. In such a place, when you lie down under a tree and look up into the spaces between the branches and wait, you will feel it. It may cause you to fall into a Neutral that makes you feel your weariness on the way into the Neutral. It may feel like dying or like you may die ... You will only pass away from suffering into beauty, emptiness, and rest. We use so much willpower that we are all weary at a level we do not perceive until it heals. At the Neutral, the stillness swallows us and we find inside it a suspending peace. An ocean. The first experience in nature of its Wholeness.

Traveling on a back road looking for the undisturbed places is a form of seeking, the pioneer in another world. Once found, these places become rest homes. An hour from my home is a lake ... all around it is this special stillness. People go there and swim. Once a certain number of visitors arrive, it is less obvious that this stillness is there. You can feel it being used up in the effort to balance the whole. After years of constant abuse, the rate changes and only Level Two Stillness is appreciated.

The "space between" was a topic that Dr. Sutherland wrote about, as did Dr. Schooley. It is a description of the landscape inside us, rather than outside in the wild. It is a skill to feel the space between rather than the anatomy when you treat. (See the year 1951 in *Contributions of Thought* and the article on Fulcrums in the 1953 *OCA Journal.*)

The meditation I described above is worth the time. It will change the way you read these writings. In 1971, I experienced this Third Level Stillness in between the forms in the woods. I remember thinking that it was God. It moved me into a spiritual study that paralleled my osteopathic interests in cranial. The two roads joined in later years.

Third Level Stillness is a meeting place. Places where we go to meet nature, meet the healing Tide, meet our Health, meet the Ocean we live in, and meet children. Children live beyond and in the landscapes of this Stillness. When we are present to this Third Level and wait with neutrality (without expectation) we will be centered by a higher presence. Here is the point of no return. We cannot use our willpower to be present. We now have a waiting place where we are met by the Tide in its infinite variety and healed in our hearts so we can be aware of the Health and its intention. This is a place where one can fool oneself into believing one is "there." It is a place that silences your reactions and creates responses in you that are welcome surprises. It is beyond comparison, beyond duality, beyond skill; it is beyond repetitions and long treatments. It is the doorway to the Master's House. Children are naturally transparent to the Health and will center us if we are at the Meeting Place.

We have studied spatial dynamics in Biodynamics of Osteopathy. We have created a language: Zone A, which is bounded by the skin; Zone B, the Fluid Body that is bounded by an area around the body; Zone C, which is a virtue; and Zone D, which is bounded by the horizon. Each zone begins from the Central Stillness and goes to the boundary referred to.

First Level Stillness is, as we have said elsewhere, the balance point of atmospheric pressure and the bodily fluids. It is found in Zone A. Second Level Stillness fills Zone B. Zone D is in the Fluid if we enter Space. The first awareness of this is in the spaces between material forms. The next level of stillness, level four, passes through everything undiminished and carries a concrete sense of holiness and love, in an ocean of infinity that is boundless. Here, one's sense of self shifts into the Divine. There is no more me and you ... All things are equally Holy. My point here is to see the dimensionality of the different levels and how each one dissolves into a greater potency and larger space.

We need to review how we came to understand these relationships.

The science of osteopathy is empirical. We watch natural laws at work and slowly begin to see relatedness. Dr. Sutherland observed for almost fifty years, and his closest students were keen and unbiased observers. One has to learn how to observe without disturbing the natural movements.

The theory of relativity says we do influence the environment. That may be true for someone with a motive, but it is possible to become invisible and not observe, but be given awareness and the facts from the environment. This happens because nature's goal is to balance everything, not just to move with indifference.

Dr. Sutherland could see phenomena, study them for years, and then ask himself, "Where's the fulcrum?" In a search for cause or a primordial fulcrum, every impression that was previously known ends, and a new place appears ... if one is too excited, tries to hold the images, or becomes fearful, then one's perception returns to the previous landscape, because one has influenced the event. The awareness of these levels comes from years of concentrated study and practice, and yet they are also given by Sutherland because, between the lines, it is all there to hear.

His lasting image of Primary Respiration is A "House Under the Sea." He attempted to say it all in one painting. The painting is lost, but not the story of his witnesses. The description of the house under the sea is reviewed elsewhere. But look at what he found, and the work he persisted in doing. Why? Well, I can only speak for myself, and guess from all the stories I have heard from his friends. Why? Because the clinical outcomes increase exponentially and one's own Health is brought closer into view. When you love something, it can open many doors for you, and the wind can clear the stale air inside. This is why. Or perhaps there is a divine plan for each of us and it persists with us until we pattern the Health in ourselves.

When we come to Second Level Stillness and it ripens our neutrality, we begin to feel the Long-Tide and its wholeness ... If perused, then one falls in love with life. After many years, one has the courage to want to see if there is more; the cause of the Long-Tide, its fulcrum, is sought ... at the risk of losing everything. This becomes a confrontation with one's own desire for power and security, which may be bridged if one loves the Mystery as a living presence, and not energy; I cannot convey how hard it is to shift one's being into a new world permanently... not for just a moment or two. The Long-Tide unfolds from a Dynamic Stillness (Third Level Stillness). This stillness is called dynamic because of its effect on the observer. As this stillness comes into view, the observer may become frightened—later, maybe aghast. Then when the observer is Neutral, the Dynamic Stillness centers one in the Divine ... one sees the Health, and no lesions.

One only sees Health. Children are seen, as they are not parented by anything other than Divine Love.

Third Level Stillness is called the Dynamic Stillness. It centers us. We begin occasionally to feel a Neutral, which has no connection to our personal will. It holds us on its center. Here, we enter a "house under the sea." We are a guest. We rest. We are served. This being served awakens a memory of innocence. One stops yearning and waits. Like a child, one becomes dependent, free of independence ... free to receive love and to begin to love others from Neutrality that is encapsulated from worldly input. These moments of wonderful purity bear no taint of one's will. It is clear that it is a gift from the Master, and a window has opened from absolute trust in his teaching and healing.

THIRD LEVEL STILLNESS

The reason we identify different kinds of stillness is because different levels come into view as we allow our mind to change. Different levels exist because our perception is lesioned. Generally, we are not aware of the laws of nature and the Breath of Life and have little discernment in these matters. Generally we are products of our education, not life.

Our study of the laws concerning Primary Respiration has awoken us to different kinds of stillness, with distinct spatial dynamics, potencies, and therapeutic tempos. This is of great help in treatment.

Normal perception can only be understood if one reads authorities on aboriginal life or mystics who have left the secular world. Most people believe that their perception is accurate, and that they are above normal. This is reflected in the projections that rule individual mental activity in our culture. The topic of normal perception should be of interest to physicians and especially traditional osteopaths. I will leave it here unless there are further inquiries as to what I understand.

Third Level Stillness is also called the Dynamic Stillness, the Meeting Place, and occasionally Natural Stillness (when in the wilderness). The variety of names given to Third Level Stillness highlight specific attributes we relate to in different areas of our teaching. To put it all under one name would accent the Mystery and weaken our understanding, which leads to the Magnitude of the Divine. We would have no trail map, and in clinical practice that is a safety issue. Third Level Stillness is native to nature. This Natural Stillness is intrinsic to wilderness settings. When we enter a wilderness, there are no roads and very few travelers. No psychic toxins from civilization. No distractions, recreation, or amusements. The air is clear, the environment unpredictable. One must pay attention and not be subservient to internal considerations. When one does this, the stillness is dynamic. It overshadows all sounds. It rules the sensory world. It echoes immortally. It frees the heart from the illusion that death is a black hole. It is a food that strengthens all atrophy. It hardens the bones.

If one is suddenly thrown into this landscape, the emptiness can be frightening. The power of the stillness, the absence of trivia, and the sense of isolation from the familiar can be fierce. Many first-time visitors are disarmed and become emotionally fragile. Some become ill. This drama is much less acute when we are learning osteopathy. The wilderness experience, however, is more intense because the entirety of the familiar is gone.

At first, experience with Third Level Stillness during treatment frightened me; I backed off quickly. I ran for something familiar. There was boundless emptiness. Any ideas of time, space, and God all disintegrated in one second. I realized I had only ideas and emotions but not a living and sustained experience of the things I believed. I slowly returned and, as a consequence, found different kinds of stillness along the way. I made a map.

Let's look at something we can do to study stillness and, in particular, Third Level Stillness.

If you travel on back roads you will find some spots where there is a Third Level Stillness. In such a place, when you step out of the vehicle you will feel a silence in the air. HERE HERE HERE

As we return to the choice to move forward and "dig on," we find, internally, a dependency upon a higher will. We can see the Dynamic Stillness centering us. Being centered by something other than oneself is so rich and purifying that the body actually begins to prefer this other will to its own, as a taskmaster. The frenzy of our self-will drives us and fools us into a sense of knowing something that elevates us. When centered by Third Level Stillness, one feels relief from the task of doing everything oneself. The indwelling peace that is effected by this power slowly changes the quality of the Neutral in us. One becomes much less judgmental of self or others. The noise of the world, and one's mental wanderings, are in another landscape that one chooses to ignore, for the purpose of remaining near one's Health.

The body continues to migrate toward this "room" inside us, and finally only the psyche remains as a barrier to choice and freedom. The psyche thrusts its sword at us, and as it does, we see who we have been. How we have seen the world and ourselves. The ego bursts into the moment trying to distract us. But it cannot enter the room. This room is neutral and inside the house under the sea. It is not ours to own or decorate. We are a guest. The love and care we receive as a guest breaks away any idea of comfort. There is love and response. Life moves from the Creator through creation. One feels begotten, anew every second that it is given to be awake to the movement of life. There is no plan. There is no intuition, no reason, and no being separate from the source. One has no posture that is from the ego. It is not a dwelling place for "experts."

It is home for the traveler who smelled its fire and went afar into the nearness.

Children are a part of the natural and the Divine. They live in a world as yet undefined by adults. They are a great and free Mystery. The indwelling therapeutics in children is beyond Third Level Stillness. This means that by using our intention, our will, we as adults cannot enter their world. As we were working to understand the issue of will that this stillness brings to us, we discovered that if we go to the shoreline of the Sea of stillness that breeds the Long-Tide, then wait there, we become a guest in the child's presence, and as such become centered by the Health shining through the child. Much has happened from this understanding that has benefited both child and us. This is why, when we talk about Third Level Stillness in Pediatrics, we call it the Meeting Place. It is a place where we are met and healed by a higher presence.

The interchanges you have with children will surprise you. I receive reports every week from osteopaths worldwide who are pleased and surprised at what transpires in difficult circumstances … if we are really there and neutral to outcomes.

OSTEOPATHIC THINKING AND THE TREATMENT OF CHILDREN

Dr. Still's writings are not arranged in a textbook, and so one must search and reread his words many times. Why do this? My reason is that every time I reread him my clinical results improve, and just as important, I better understand why he and we need a separate profession from the mainstream of Western medicine.

In *Philosophy of Osteopathy* he writes about the basic principles he uses in thinking osteopathy. He was not a structuralist, by his own admission. He considered the whole patient a living reality and sought to establish that wholeness. His vision was that when wholeness was present, all the fluids were free and in abundance. In this state a patient would heal without drugs or remedies other than God's built-in drugstore. The state of disease was in the patient's mind, the outcome of stasis, fermentation, and putrefaction. Once the "withering field" was refreshed, the patient would heal. His success rate in treating infectious diseases made him well respected and sought after as a clinician.

"Think osteopathy rather than thinking osteopathically" are the words Sutherland chose to highlight the two streams of thought in our culture. I will not belabor this point. It is, however, crucial to understanding children and interactions with them.

Sutherland also calls upon us to use our imagination with a capital "I." Osteopathic thinking is not what most osteopaths do.

Osteopathic thinking, as described by our founder and his intimate followers, is divergent thinking. It is thinking independently of what you know. One thinks with an empty mind. There is no cause that is arrived at reductionistically. Cause is met with the thinking, knowing, and feeling hands that are connected, not to a textbook, but to the Health of the patient and a history directed away from the allopathic ideas and toward the whole and its moment of compromise.

Thinking osteopathy is a science of divergence ... thinking away from the known into the movement of the unknown, bringing it into the foreground for a moment and then letting it pass. This kind of activity is toward the whole patient—not the cause of the symptoms. It embraces stillness in the center of the process.

There are books on this subject. Or you can watch children! Intelligence is not really about a graduate education.

Convergent thinking is the norm for adults. It is thinking that moves toward a predetermined goal, which is set in the reduction of data into a format, or a belief, or bias. Convergent thinking is closed before it starts. It fires imagination. It is dependent on the known facts. It is not reason. It is not imagination. Both reason and imagination are higher functions. Dr. Still saw reason as a divine wisdom, a gift ... as did Aristotle.

Divergent thinking moves away from any predetermined goal. It is open to the "not yet" that is coming in the moment of being. It is not afraid of inadequacies or failure, nor is it bold. It is open and not reductionistic. It is creative within the movements of life, not one's past knowledge. Unlike convergence, it is patient, neutral, and does not lead the patient or jump to conclusions. It sees the Whole.

This process includes diagnosis and history, brought to a point of meaningfulness by the Health in both parties. It is often curative as it happens. The chief complaint is a doorway into a story of how the functional reserve in the whole became compromised. The parts follow a larger picture; they do not lead it.

This is how it is with children ...

Children can really help us undo our convergence. But we must meet them on their landscape. And with adults like Drs. Still, Sutherland, Wales, Becker, Day, Laughlin, Johnston … et cetera.

Recommended reading and viewing:

1. *Philosophy of Osteopathy,* Andrew Taylor Still D.O. … it is a small book. How does he want us to think?
2. "The Tour of the Minnow" … last article in *Contributions of Thought,* William Garner Sutherland D.O.
3. Oxford English Dictionary, Unabridged … see definition for "Imagination"
4. *The Spiritual Life of Children,* Robert Coles
5. Ken Robinson RSA, YouTube.com. Several videos with great discussions on children and divergent thinking
6. The selected writings of Beryl E. Arbuckle D.O.

BRAIN SAG

At eighty-six years of age, Dr. Still climbed a tree.

The aging process, as seen by the allopathic profession, is that elders are ready to be recycled. It is not unusual for elders to be seen as children and treated that way.

Many of our teachers lived strong, vivid lives, right to the moment of Dawn.

Osteopathy can prevent much decline in the aging soma. Today we will study one.

We all have heard of sacral sag, where the sacrum feels hard and is unable to rise vertically or respond to either of the two respirations. Sag means a "withering field" and the loss of vertical height in a function of the Fluid Body. This can occur at any age. Some sags that are common:

Sacral sag

Diaphragmatic sag, with stress on the kidneys and resultant moderate hypertension and dependent edema

Thoracic spine kyphosis and loss of tallness; secondary osteoporosis

Lower arch sag of the foot with aggravation or promotion of pelvic floor sag

All of these need reestablishment of fluid dynamics ... i.e., until the vertical height returns ... and the feel of sag is gone.

The hallmark symptoms are a general slowing of all faculties: vitality, enthusiasm, mental acuity, appetite, etc. ... One would think, "Mom is getting a little senile," and the doctor might agree.

The brain MRI shows that the cerebellum is low and the cisterna magnum is shallow (loss of vertical height). The diagnosis is confirmed, but there is no treatment. It's called aging!

The brain sag is easy to treat with good results.

In pregnant women, morning sickness seems to be related to a functional brain sag that is easily addressed.

BOWL OF WATER

Practical

Hold the head like a bowl of water in the ocean.
Make sure the neck muscles are in Neutral.
Notice the position of the cerebellum and the height of the waterbed upon which it rests; is it buoyant?
Is there a response in the cerebellum and the waterbed to Thoracic Respiration?
To Primary Respiration?
Does the fluid internally disengage and transmute in response to the Tide?
Go to the Dynamic Stillness in the fluid
... Wait
When Thoracic Respiration begins moving the fluid and the cerebellum, the Tide will be coming shortly. Then the cerebellum floats like a cork in the ocean.
Let the patient rest; when they are aroused again, check the need for rebalancing.
Rebalancing: Zone B and the "sea around us," moving as one.

THE MOVING CHILD

The Meeting Place is a wonderful and deeply alive room. It is in all of us. Children know it well.

Adults have left this place behind in search of success, both in the world and in themselves.

The Meeting Place is where we, as adults, enter into a room inside us where we become aware of the shoreline of an ocean of love and eternity. It is the doorway to the Health.

Children are more perceptive than adults. This fact places us at a lower level of awareness than a child. This means that any attempt to control them must be sanctioned by the child.

Poorly behaved children are usually the product of specific aging processes that challenge them, like the two- or three-year-old child that commonly says "no" a lot. These children are not difficult to "meet" if we have an inner commitment to staying at the Meeting Place and not being distracted or frustrated by our desire to achieve "control" of them.

Other children appear "hyperactive" but settle into the Meeting Place once they realize an adult can be trusted in a manner that is real for them; an instinctual awareness of inner peace in the adult makes a child feel safe. Why? Well, most adults are treating children in such a way as to not change their adult habits, habits which are often the product of immaturity in the adult. Adults are generally unaware of a child's inner world.

When you, as a practitioner, remain at the Meeting Place, you will feel no inner tension or need to change any child's behavior, unless, of course, it is destructive.

The Meeting Place has become a special place to meet Life and the Tide. In the wave of one comes an opening that children know well.

The interchanges you have with children will surprise you. I receive reports every week from osteopaths worldwide who are pleased and surprised at what transpires in difficult circumstances, if we are really there and neutral to outcomes.

For thou hast possessed my reins: thou hast covered me in my mother's womb.

I will praise thee; for I am fearfully and wonderfully made: marvellous are thy works; and that my soul knoweth right well.

My substance was not hid from thee, when I was made in secret, and curiously wrought in the lowest parts of the earth.

Thine eyes did see my substance, yet being unperfect; and in thy book all my members were written, which in continuance were fashioned, when as yet there was none of them.

Psalm 139:13–16, KJV

A CHILD'S SENSE OF WHOLENESS

Children's experience of Wholeness is alive. For adults, the memory of this is limp.

Children feel a family circle and are intent on being in it. They bring the adults into it, and a new Zone B is felt by the adults that transcends the individual Zone B. We will discuss this as a topic and as a practical.

Children are normally aware of things many adults search for.

When you treat, hold the child's sense of Wholeness in your heart. Let it lead you on to your own recollection and the spatial dynamics of the child's awareness.

Children also know the oneness of the spiritual family, formed by all children. They even have a universal language. From this understanding, adults can begin to feel this also.

When we treat a particular child and are aware of all the children who will never be treated, who have no access to help, then we open a doorway to seeing into their world a little.

There is plenty of love in the "mechanism" for everyone. Do not crowd the awareness of a child. They can lead you without dismissing your help and treatment.

Do not put old wine in new bottles.

What Is the Child Looking at in You?

BIODYNAMICS OF OSTEOPATHY BOOK SERIES

This book is one of a series of twelve *Biodynamics of Osteopathy* books. It is recommended that you read the whole series in order, as each book builds on the understanding from prior books. It is also recommended that you seek experienced teachers and mentors to help you experience the full depth of the information given.

The full series is as follows:

Phase One is about involuntary motion, which is motion present in the whole and in the lesion. We learn to synchronize with the breathing of Primary Respiration before we approach any treatment. This synchronization is the key to working with stable rates and not irritating the system. The principle of synchronizing with a healthy aspect of the patient suffuses the whole teaching program. This synchronization shifts our awareness to a different level of receptivity, which allows us to see Primary Respiration rather than the lesion field, and this eventually leads us to an understanding of the intention of Primary Respiration.

Phase Two is about communication with the natural laws of healing that surround activity at 2 to 3 cycles per minute. We synchronize with the breathing of Primary Respiration and also add the skill of sensing the fulcrum, the Stillness through which the breathing creates form and function. It is a different kind of synchronization from that in Phase One, shifting our awareness more deeply. As this occurs, the treatment automatically expresses itself. The end point of treatment, when compared with Phase One, reveals several differences. We find this kind of synchronization works exclusively with the fluid body and the outcome of treatment is more complete than when working with tissue alone.

Phase Three is centered around the activities of the Long Tide (100 second cycle). We explore an indwelling therapeutic force already present in the lesion field. We learn that the dural system is not made-up of three sickles but rather a series of folds in a sac, arising during growth and development. We see the relationship between the upper and lower dural sacs, awakening us to the independence of two separate tentorium cerebelli. We discover that zone D, the horizon, and the Wire (along which the Long Tide moves during its intended therapeutic course) are all linked as natural laws pertaining to this level of Primary Respiration.

Phase Four focuses on the Midline, a place where the spatial relationships are expressed as a whole. It synchronizes and centers us in such a way that we become aware of Zone D and the Dynamic Stillness. The Third Level Stillness in Phase Four is different from the Stillness in the other Phases – we are centered by the Stillness at the center of creation. Our intention is replaced by the intention of the Tide which can facilitate our spiritual path.

Phase Five is about *the face*. As we approach the face, we use all of the principles that we have learned in Phase One, Two, Three, and Four. We work with automatic shifting and notice differences from how the face is viewed by older models within Osteopathy in the Cranial Field. As we synchronize with the therapeutic presence of the Long Tide we see what we can learn about the face from that landscape. We also work with Seams, Dynamic Stillness, and Ignition.

Phase Six is a continuation of our journey into the Wholeness that generates life and delivers therapeutic forces that transmute lesions once Neutral is expressed. It is a mixture of activities centered around the outside presence of Primary Respiration as something that is a non-biological force and that has a persona. We will also continue to explore seams and then move on to the extremities, first in the embryological terms and then as Sutherland taught them in his work called PowerPoints. Phase 6 is a time to build your understanding of the Tide and refine your skills.

Phase Seven highlights the Health. Dr. Still's famous comment "Find the Health; anyone can find disease," has plagued many minds over the last century. We come to the clear vision of several indwelling aspects of the Health: Love ... liquid light ... and a diamond matrix. A approach to the terminally ill and dying patient is addressed. In the somatic sensation of the Tide passing through the House Under the Sea, our awareness is transmuted by the Health. The lesion is seen as a precognitive act of the Health. Thoracic Respiration, Primary Respiration, and Ignition are as One. The landscape is vast ... and the principles of healing are even more substantial than we have previously experienced..

Phase Eight is a deeper exploration of seams, balanced rhythmic interchange, and the Flame of Intention as a therapeutic modality. Phase Eight is the culmination of our awareness of Wholeness, and ultimately brings us to the Divine Presence, Unconditional Love and Oneness. The living Tide dominates the awareness while forms move to the background. One feels the Breath of Creation in oneself as the Center of Wholeness. One feels the Unfoldment of oneself as one is Created. Our consciousness is a gift; we do not own it and if we try to control it we lose Wholeness.

Phase Nine is when we are able to fully evaluate and treat the

Central Nervous System and the Eye. We also address Fire and the therapeutic modality of the Shakedown. True action is moved from Love and makes our perception exist. This Love is self-emptying and by its nature allows us to Serve as part of the Perfect. Perception can be used to Serve something other than ourselves. We have attempted to enter this balance point between the Perfect and the Disease ... it is a point where the whole of everything is suspended by Love as it works to incarnate the Complete. In the balance point of everything is The Intention of the Tide following the movement of the distortion back to a True relationship with the Blueprint of Life.

Pediatrics One explores how children grow as a whole, not in parts as we sometimes believe. Children live in the Direction of Ease of motion present in their fluid metabolic fields, otherwise they get uncomfortable and require assistance. Does your treatment directly support the whole, or does it assume to support the whole? We realize children are not adults and cannot be treated as adults are. We approach the therapeutic modality of the "Meeting Place", prenatal and postnatal periods, the treatment of the pelvis during pregnancy, fetal malposition and labor.

Pediatrics Two is where we deepen in the perceptive awareness necessary to approach the treatment of children. We deepen in our appreciation of Wholeness, the three levels of Stillness and the "Meeting Place". We approach "Desert Neutral", where therapeutics pass into the neutral substance, and a mystery unfolds as the breath of Divine love cascades as a therapeutic force across a night desert landscape, filling and leaving behind no visible effects. We further address treatment of the pelvis and the uterus during pregnancy. We explore thoracic and Primary Respiration in children, and the Family Circle.

Pediatrics Three is where we continue to study the therapeutic

Flow of Attention. We deepen in Third Level Stillness and the Meeting Place. The Meeting Place is easily misinterpreted … our observer must be so still and neutral that the process can be seen as it happens. The central nervous system in the child can be finally approached for evaluation and treatment. We explore teething and also the "locked up head". We use the therapeutic modality of the Flame of Intention, and its connection to the Breath of Life. Everything is transparent to the Breath of Life.

ABOUT THE AUTHOR

James Jealous, D.O. (1943–2021), was an osteopathic physician, teacher, and writer. His life's work was founding and developing **Biodynamics of Osteopathy**, a unique methodology he established within the field of osteopathy, following the lineage of Dr. A.T. Still and Dr. W.G. Sutherland.

He was born in Saco, Maine, and since his father was an osteopathic physician, he was around osteopathy from an early age. He studied at Kirksville College of Osteopathic Medicine in Missouri (now the A.T. Still University of Health Sciences), graduating in 1970. He then set up practice in rural Maine as an osteopathic primary care physician.

Over time, Dr. Jealous saw parallels between the work of embryologist Dr. Erich Blechschmidt and that of osteopathic physician Dr. William Garner Sutherland. This inspiration led him to create his own body of work. In the early 1990s, he began teaching "A Biodynamic View of Osteopathy in the Cranial Field," which, as he developed his specific methodology, was refined to "Biodynamics of Osteopathy."

A deeply spiritual person, he felt most at home in the natural world and was an avid fisherman and hiker.

For more information, please visit:
https://BiodynamicsOfOsteopathy.com

There is a wind passing through …
it is the motion of creation,
the eternal motion of Divine love.